HOW TO CREATE AN AMAZING BRAIN

10 ways to keep your brain sharp as you age

By

Mortimer Jerome Adler

Table of content
Introduction

Conclusion

Introduction

Rather a good place to focus on your brain-building goals is in focus. From what we can see or prove, the cognitive domain of attention is unquestionably the most adaptable.

Even if you only spend a few minutes concentrating on your breath, meditation is a good way to strengthen your brain.

At the point when individuals ponder, throughout the span of weeks their hippocampus develops, their prefrontal cortex expands in volume, and their trepidation locator the amygdala of possible psychologists.

Because you can't focus when you are anxious or stressed, that last part is crucial.

Brain cells are toxic to cortisol.

Meditation can help you get out of the fight or flight mode, but you can't get rid of all your stress.

Although brain scans of some 70 year olds are comparable to those of 20 to 30 year olds, important parts of the brain tend to shrink as we get older.

Research suggests routines that might help keep the mind sharp as we get older.

Cognitive decline is not inevitable as you get older, contrary to popular belief and adopting healthy habits can significantly lower your risk of developing dementia in later life.

People almost always have the ability to think more creatively, according to research, and those effects are significant and repeatable. In neuroscience, Green cites the cells that fire together, wire together age-old adage.

The idea is that the connections between the cells involved become stronger the more you use your brain to do something.

We all experience anxiety from time to time, it is a perfectly normal, healthy response meant to protect us.

Anxiety originates in the part of the brain that anticipates trouble and prepares us to fight or flee in response to it.

Threats can also include humiliation, shame, separation from a loved one, missing out, and not being able to do something you want to do.

This can make it really hard to avoid anything that makes you anxious.

That avoidance will sometimes make sense, but it can also cause us to avoid things that would actually be good for us at times. The good news is that this can be circumvented.

Regardless, the strategies listed below are not only well worth your time and effort but also have been shown to enhance information processing, concentration, memory, and storage of your brain.

Chapter 1

How the brain works.

Where does creativity reside in the brain?

A specific address in the brain is the source of some bodily functions, like wagging one's toes.
However, creativity is more like a floating boat than a static street address. It includes mind networks connecting memory and language, spatial comprehension, and fine coordinated abilities.

The creative party boat floats down the networks, which are analogous to rivers that are interconnected. Ordinary barges also use these rivers to solve math problems, follow recipes, and read reports.
However, creativity is not as mysterious as it may initially appear. There are two ways your brain can help you come up with a creative idea through more critical thinking and the well known "aha" moment of insight. Even when you sleep, daydream, or relax, your brain still solves difficult problems, and aha moments depend on unconscious mental processes.

When you move around or are in a slightly disoriented state, you might get a great insight. Because of this, it might come to you while you're in the shower, on a walk, or even at 2 a.m.

Creativity can also come from carefully analyzing and solving problems step by step. You can end up with something completely novel if you consciously invent, tinker, evaluate, and modify ideas.

Additionally, your ability to solve problems will improve, allowing you to better navigate the world and improve your health.

Therefore, while creativity provides its own reward and may encourage your child to eat her broccoli, it also contributes to the health of your brain as a whole.

Over the past 15 years, a growing number of arts organizations and studies have discovered that participating in creative endeavors can help prevent loneliness, reduce dementia, and increase engagement.

Conversely, cognitive decline may accelerate when we are not exposed to anything new.

Any activity that keeps the brain active aids in aging, when we grow new brain cells and make new connections between the ones we already have when we take on new hobbies, learn new skills, or deal with new situations. Painting, writing, math, or learning a language are all examples of creative experiences that stimulate brain cells.

Art therapy, writing therapy, and other forms of creative expression may be uplifting and effective for many people because creativity can activate the brain's reward system. It is just not true that we think we are not creative.

Creativity can be as simple as walking in a certain way or doing a little dance when you get good news. You are creative.

Chapter 2

Experiences teaches the brain

The more you avoid something, the more you teach your brain that the only way to feel safe is to avoid that situation. On the other hand, the more you bravely do something, the more you teach your brain that you are okay even if you are anxious.

Using a tool known as a stepladder is one way to retrain your brain to cope with anxiety. The plan is to gradually progress through experiences that make you more anxious until you can do what you've been avoiding.

Let's say for instance, that social situations give you anxiety.

Create a stepladder by starting with a social situation that makes you feel a little anxious and working your way up to steps that get harder slowly and gently.

Going out with your family to a new location might be a good way to start your step ladder. You may experience some anxiety as a result, but it is manageable.

Repeat that several times until you feel comfortable with it. After that, proceed to the following ladder step. This might be going somewhere a friend is familiar with.

The following step might bc to go somewhere new with a few friends.

You are completely in charge of the steps. Repeat each step as many times as necessary until you feel comfortable. It's usually a sign that there is too much distance between the steps if one of them makes you feel like your anxiety is going to explode. Until you are ready to move on to the next step, simply return to something that feels a little safer.

Your brain is being taught that you are safe even when you feel anxious by every step you take. You can stay on a particular step for weeks or months because there is no rush to complete any of the steps. Until you are ready to move on to the next step, take as long as necessary, you can actually re-teach your brain that you are safe, that you can get through this, and that you don't have to avoid the situations that make you anxious by gradually exposing yourself to them.

You will be surprised at what you can accomplish if you are patient and gentle with yourself during the process. Similar to how a crutch might help you walk if you broke your leg, compensatory strategies are workarounds that help you complete tasks.

Think back to the song you sang to remember the presidents, or how you imagined a hydrant with a balloon attached to remind you that hydrogen and helium start the periodic table.

The majority of the things you can do to improve your memory are things like making it a habit to hang your car keys on a hook by the door and repeating a new person's name when you meet them.

However, only a small number of cognitive rehabilitation techniques are restorative, indicating that they actually repair or enhance brain function.

Consider for instance, how a stroke victim might need to relearn how to walk or speak. In addition, you can improve your recall and comprehension, focus your memory, and perform other tasks that are related to brain health by engaging in other healthy habits like getting enough sleep and eating well.

When you expect to improve your brain function, what should you anticipate? What people are willing to do determines what is realistic.

Even though some brain training is enjoyable, not all of it is. You get out of it what you put into it, much like with diet and exercise.

Chapter 3

How to achieve brain training work

Brain training: What is it? When we learn, what happens?

Brain training is an easy but effective way to improve a student's fundamental ability to learn more quickly, easily, and effectively. Through a complex network of nerve cells called neurons, the brain processes information. Groups of neurons physically collaborate to complete learning or thinking tasks as we learn.

According to research, when the task is novel or unfamiliar or when the learning demand is increased, additional nearby neurons are drawn into this process.

The borrowed neurons are released to return to other tasks after the task is completed, nonetheless, the additions in productivity and handling speed expected for that undertaking are held and make learning related errands simpler.

Cognitive training also known as brain training is a non pharmacological strategy that entails performing a series of regular mental activities to help a person maintain or even improve their cognitive (thinking) abilities.

Additionally, there are more general kinds of mental training that can aid in maintaining or enhancing cognitive fitness. Similar to how exercise improves and maintains physical health, this more general mental training focuses on maintaining the brain's fitness.

Brain adaptability characterizes the cerebrum capacity to change and adjust neuron action and associations in response to expanded learning interest.

Gray matter can actually thin out or thicken up, and neural connections can be made, improved or conversely weakened by certain activities in the environment. Brain training makes use of neuroplasticity by putting a student through specially designed exercises that help these neuronal connections grow and strengthen quickly.

With the right training, cognitive abilities like memory, attention, sensory processing, and reasoning can be improved. This makes the brain work better now and in the future, improves recall, speeds up processing, and makes learning a lot easier for a wide range of learning challenges.

Individual cognitive abilities like auditory and visual processing and memory are honed through brain training when information is transformed into knowledge. Different learning difficulties necessitate different skill combinations.

Learning that is based on a particular skill will be hindered if required skills are lacking. Brain training has the power to identify, target and then strengthen individual cognitive skills through testing. Individual training exercises speed up and make learning easier by strengthening particular skills.

The brain never stops changing, as research has shown. Brain training may be your best option if you or your child are having difficulty learning to read or write and want to move on to reading and writing success.

There are two types of strategies used to improve cognitive skills in the field of cognitive rehabilitation that are typically focused on stroke or brain injury patients which are rehabilitative and compensatory.

Additionally, they are adaptable to the rest of us.

Chapter 4

Put Your Mind to the Test.

Learning new skills and engaging in other mentally stimulating activities can assist your brain in becoming more adaptable and adjusting to changes brought on by aging.

Challenging your brain is thought to activate processes that help maintain individual brain cells and stimulate communication between them. Your brain is more engaged the more senses you use. Try a new style of music or a new cuisine. Make lifelong learning a priority because brain connection building and preservation are ongoing processes.

Chapter 5

Stay Connected

Social connections aids in reducing feelings of depression and isolation. Engage in activities that are important to you. Volunteering, being a part of your community and spending time with friends and family are all options.

Being around other people has a positive emotional impact on many people and ageing is a time of loss and adjustment for many. Additionally, it has the potential to improve relationships, enliven the spirit, and stimulate the brain. It is so important to keep in touch with other people.

However, the key is making more time in your day for active thinking, usually by disconnecting from email, social media, and other sources. That is how to get to the digressive, slow, uncertain parts of ourselves that are key to our creativity. Try incorporating this idea into your daily routine by not taking your phone to bed or the bathroom.

Notification settings for email and social media apps should also be disabled. Before any brainstorming session, you should think about making a specific time in your day for creative thinking and remind yourself to do so.

Chapter 6

How to train your brain

Have you ever lost it at work and then deeply regretted your actions or words later?.

Have you felt so deeply insulted or hurt that it hampered your performance at work?. Both cases reflect that you were out of control and were being dictated by either your reptilian or emotional brain while your logical brain was imprisoned.

Research states that our brain has three independent regions which are the reptilian, the limbic or emotional brain and the neocortex or cognitive brain and they all control our thoughts, behaviour or action.

Your reptilian brain evolved and matured over 200 million years ago. It deals with survival and reproduction and triggers anger, stress fight or flight response. It also has no sense of language or time.

Your limbic system or the paleo-mammalian brain evolved with the first mammals and it deals with sensory information and assigns emotions to events, thus controlling your emotions.

It operates in the present and is motivated only by pleasure and pain, like experiencing negative feelings when colleagues criticise you. The neocortex or the task-oriented region of your brain evolved from higher mammals and gives you language, perception, planning and abstraction. It also gets you ahead in your career by helping you stay in control.

The three regions of your brain work independently on three tasks namely survive, enjoy and thrive. When you are thinking about survival or are only enjoying the present and avoiding the pain, you cannot thrive or succeed in your career.

Your crocodile or dinosaur brain has triggers ranging from fear and survival including financial security. At work, irrational fears about your boss or losing your job can trigger your survival response causing you to fight or run away.

Your emotional brain also has triggers, so when you avoid the pain of tough learning assignments at work and choose the immediate pleasure of browsing the Internet instead of finishing your project, your emotional brain is in control.

When at work, if you find yourself tilting towards irrational anger or violence in a charged situation, practice slowing down.

Observe what is happening in your body either tightness of breath and muscle or an accelerated pulse rate.

Instead of reacting, focus on consciously slowing down your breathing. If that doesn't give immediate results, go for a brisk walk to work off the stress.

Let your cognitive brain take control. In case your colleague is seized by his reptilian brain and has started abusing, choose to walk away and return when the situation has calmed down your brain instead of overworking it.

Chapter 7

Start making friends.

Social isolation increases dementia risk by 50% in older adults. The connection is obvious. However, you are not required to gather an entire group of companions, a handful of close friends can suffice.

Spend more time with your neighbors, volunteer at a community center, or adopt a pet, for example, rather than trying to make as many friends as you can, concentrate on creating the social networks that best suit your needs.

Hearing loss is a common ageing issue that can make it difficult to socialize.

Although addressing hearing loss is essential to brain health, social withdrawal may be easier than confronting embarrassment over hearing loss and working to correct it.

For every 10-decibel loss of hearing, cognitive performance decreases, stress from loneliness also raises cortisol levels which may harm the brain over time.

Chapter 8

Relax, Stress is a normal part of life.

Stress that you can manage, which challenges you, motivates you, and helps you grow actually helps your brain.

However, relaxation is just as important.

Meditation practitioners have thicker brain regions associated with focus and attention. Music is another great stress reliever because it can be performed and enjoyed with friends, which may increase its impact on cognitive longevity to its fullest extent.

A good night's sleep is one way that relaxation helps keep your mind sharp.

Memories can only be stored and consolidated in deep sleep. Adults who sleep poorly over time are more likely to develop Alzheimer's disease symptoms.

However, simple routines such as limiting food and drink three hours before bedtime, maintaining the same sleep schedule, and not looking at smartphones or other electronic devices in the bedroom, can improve sleep at any age.

Chapter 9

Staying physically active.

This is one of the best ways to maintain youthfulness as the body ages. The brain is the same way. If there is one thing you can do to improve your brain health, it is exercise. The evidence is overwhelming.

Exercise raises a protein known as brain-derived neurotrophic factor, which is necessary for the growth and maintenance of neurons. Among other benefits, exercise also helps prevent inflammation in the brain. Every week, try to get 150 minutes of aerobic exercise and one to two days of strength training.

Exercise also reduces mental stress and lowers risk factors for dementia such as high blood pressure, diabetes, and high cholesterol. Regular muscle-building exercises like walking quickly, doing squats or lunges, or lifting hand weights are all good options.

Regardless of your age, eating well and getting enough sleep are good habits everyone should adopt. Also, if you smoke, quit. A healthy way of life benefits your mind and body at the same time.
If you combine exercise with other healthy strategies, the benefits may increase.

Try adding a cognitive challenge, like dancing or playing sports, which combine music, socializing, a cardio workout, and learning the steps. In like manner, yoga might help mind wellbeing since it joins reflection with development.

Another benefit may come from exercising outside in the fresh air by reducing stress and increasing melatonin. Exposure to natural light and greenery promotes a more regular sleep-wake cycle, both of which are beneficial to brain health.

Chapter 10

Choose a meal that is good for your brain

After exercising, such as berries and green leafy vegetables, which are important for brain health. These diets will improve cardiovascular health, which can also protect the brain.

Changing the microbiome, a collection of trillions of bacteria that live in the gut and influence the health of many parts of the body, can also change the composition of people's blood pressure, which has been linked to a lower risk of Alzheimer's disease.

27

Conclusion

The evidence that brain training will assist you in becoming smarter is at best mixed, despite the fact that your developing brain is extremely flexible and it ought to be possible to do so.

Multiple activities that are based on actual situations are likely to be included in future brain training programs. However, do not wait for brand new programs.

If you want to improve on how your brain is going to work, do something today to stay active, eat healthy, get enough sleep, and keep learning new things by reading a lot.

Congratulations, you are already doing it.

Printed in Great Britain
by Amazon